MW01601278

GAPS DIET

MAIN COURSE – 80 + Quick and easy to prepare at home recipes to heal your GUT and boost digestive health

TABLE OF CONTENTS

☞Copyright 2018 by Noah Jerris - All rights reserved.

This document is geared towards providing exact and reliable information in regards to the topic and issue covered. The publication is sold with the idea that the publisher is not required to render accounting, officially permitted, or otherwise, qualified services. If advice is necessary, legal or professional, a practiced individual in the profession should be ordered.

- From a Declaration of Principles which was accepted and approved equally by a Committee of the American Bar Association and a Committee of Publishers and Associations.

In no way is it legal to reproduce, duplicate, or transmit any part of this document in either electronic means or in printed format. Recording of this publication is strictly prohibited and any storage of this document is not allowed unless with written permission from the publisher. All rights reserved.

The information provided herein is stated to be truthful and consistent, in that any liability, in terms of inattention or otherwise, by any usage or abuse of any policies, processes, or directions contained within is the solitary and utter responsibility of the recipient reader. Under no circumstances will any legal responsibility or blame be held against the publisher for any reparation, damages, or monetary loss due to the information herein, either directly or indirectly.

Respective authors own all copyrights not held by the publisher.

The information herein is offered for informational purposes solely, and is universal as so. The presentation of the information is without contract or any type of guarantee assurance.

The trademarks that are used are without any consent, and the publication of the trademark is without permission or backing by the trademark owner. All trademarks and brands within this book are for clarifying purposes only and are the owned by the owners themselves, not affiliated with this document.

Introduction

GAPS recipes for personal enjoyment but also for family enjoyment. You will love them for sure for how easy it is to prepare them.

BREAKFAST

BREAKFAST HASH

Serves: **6**

Prep Time: **10**   Minutes

Cook Time: **6**   Hours

Total Time: **6**   Hours 10 Minutes

INGREDIENTS

- 10 oz. sausage (GAPS Legal)
- 1 cup onion
- 1 lb. celery root
- ¼ cup thyme
- 1 bell pepper
- ½ cup chicken broth
- ¼ tsp black pepper
- parsley

DIRECTIONS

1. In a slow cooker add celery root, peppers, thyme, onion and pepper
2. Add chicken broth and cook for 4-6 hours on low, remove and serve

Serves: **6**

Prep Time: **5**   Minutes

Cook Time: **5**   Minutes

Total Time: **10**   Minutes

INGREDIENTS

- 4 eggs
- ¼ cup shredded cheese
- ½ cup onion
- ½ tsp salt

DIRECTIONS

1. Grease your waffle iron with oil
2. Crack eggs into a bowl and whisk to combine
3. Stir in cheese, salt, and onions
4. Pour mixture into waffle iron and cook for 3-4 minutes or until ready
5. Remove and serve

Serves: *8*
Prep Time: *5*   Minutes

Cook Time: *10*   Minutes

Total Time: *15*   Minutes

INGREDIENTS

- 1 cup cauliflower
- 1/3 tsp black pepper
- 1/3 cup cheddar cheese
- 1 egg
- 1 tablespoon parsley
- 1 cup carrot
- ½ cup bell pepper
- 1 cup almond flour
- 1/3 tsp salt

DIRECTIONS

1. In a bowl mix bell pepper, almond flour, salt, pepper, carrots, cauliflower
2. Add eggs, cheese and mix well

3. Pour mixture into a skillet and cook for 2-3 minutes per side or until golden brown

4. Remove and serve

PUMPKIN WAFFLES

Serves: *8*
Prep Time: *5*   Minutes

Cook Time: *10*   Minutes

Total Time: *15*   Minutes

INGREDIENTS

- 4 eggs
- 1 cup pumpkin puree
- ½ cup honey
- ½ cup coconut oil
- 1 tsp vanilla
- 2 cup cashews
- ½ cup coconut flour
- 1 cup baking soda
- ½ cup salt

- 2 tsp cinnamon
- 1 tsp ginger
- ½ tsp nutmeg
-

DIRECTIONS

1. In a blender add all ingredients and blend until smooth
2. Heat your waffle iron and pour the batter
3. Cook for 2-3 minutes or until ready
4. Remove and serve

Serves: *8*

Prep Time: *5*   Minutes

Cook Time: *10*   Minutes

Total Time: *15*   Minutes

INGREDIENTS
- 1 tablespoon butter
- 1 tablespoon honey
- 3 eggs
- 3 tablespoons coconut flour
- ¼ cup coconut milk
- 1 tsp baking soda
- 1 tsp vanilla

DIRECTIONS

1. In a bowl mix butter and honey
2. In another bowl mix egg whites and add yolks to the butter mixture
3. Add almond flour, vanilla, baking soda and mix well
4. Fold the egg whites into the pancake mixture and pour batter into a skillet and cook for 2-3 minutes
5. Remove, top with berries and serve

Serves: *4*
Prep Time: *10*   Minutes

Cook Time: *55*   Minutes

Total Time: *65*   Minutes

INGREDIENTS

- 14 oz. spinach
- ½ cup cheddar cheese
- 1 lb. yogurt
- 3 eggs
- 2 tablespoons almond flour
- ¼ tsp salt
- ¼ tsp pepper
- ¼ tsp dill
- 2 tablespoons butter
- ¼ onion
- 1/3 cup parmesan cheese

DIRECTIONS

1. **Preheat oven to 325 F**

2. In a bowl mix almond flour, pepper, dill, eggs and spinach
3. In the skillet sauté onions until tender
4. Pour in the spinach mixture and cook for 3-4 minutes
5. Remove, add parmesan cheese and bake for 50-55 minutes
6. Remove and serve

BLUEBERRY MUFFINS

Serves: *10*
Prep Time: *10* Minutes

Cook Time: *10* Minutes

Total Time: *20* Minutes

INGREDIENTS

- 2 cups almond flour
- ½ cup flaxseed meal
- ¼ cup salt
- 1 tsp baking soda
- 2 eggs

- ¼ cup honey
- ½ cup butter
- 2 tablespoons water
- 1/3 cup blueberries

DIRECTIONS

1. Preheat oven to 325 F
2. In a bowl mix honey, butter and cream with a mixer
3. Add water, eggs and the rest of dry ingredients, beat until well combined
4. Fill muffin tin cups with 2/3 and sprinkle blueberries, bake for 15-20 minutes
5. Remove and serve

Serves: **2**

Prep Time: **5**   Minutes

Cook Time: **10** Minutes

Total Time: **15** Minutes

INGREDIENTS
- 1 apple
- 1 tablespoon butter
- 1 tablespoons pecans
- ¼ tsp cinnamon
- 3 eggs
- 1 tsp
- honey

DIRECTIONS

1. Slice the apples and sprinkle cinnamon
2. Sauté for 3-4 minutes, add pecans and cook for another 2-3 minutes
3. In a bowl beat eggs and pour into another skillet and cook
4. Flip omelet over and top with apples and pecans
5. Remove and serve

Serves: *6*
Prep Time: *10*   Minutes

Cook Time: *6*   Hours

Total Time: *6*   Hours 10 Minutes

INGREDIENTS

- 12 oz. spinach
- 1 tablespoon butter
- 1 cup mushrooms
- 1 red bell pepper
- 1 cup cheddar cheese
- 6 eggs
-
- 1 tablespoon chives
- ¼ tsp salt
- ¼ cup almond flour
- ½ tsp baking soda

DIRECTIONS

1. **In a skillet heat butter over medium heat, sauté mushrooms and pepper for about 3-4 minutes**

2. In a bowl mix salt, pepper, eggs, chives, and cheese
3. Add to the egg mixture baking soda and almond flour
4. Pour everything into a slow cooker and cook on low for 4-6 hours, remove and serve

SAUSAGE EGG

Serves:	*4*	
Prep Time:	*10*	Minutes
Cook Time:	*30*	Minutes
Total Time:	*40*	Minutes

INGREDIENTS

- 1 tablespoon ghee
- ½ lb. pork sausage
- 1 egg
- salt
- black pepper
- ½ cup water
- 1 tablespoon guacamole

DIRECTIONS

1. Place a biscuit cutter on a cutting board and fill with sausage meat

2. Heat a skillet over medium heat and fry the sausage for 2-3 minutes per side

3. Beat the egg and pour into the biscuit cutter in the pan and cook until ready

4. Assemble by placing firstly the egg, meat, and guacamole and serve

Serves: **6**

Prep Time: **10** Minutes

Cook Time: **10** Minutes

Total Time: **20** Minutes

INGREDIENTS

- 3 tablespoons coconut oil
- 3 tablespoons honey
- 1 tablespoon cinnamon
- 1 tsp salt
- 3 cups cauliflower
- 3 cups milk
- 3 eggs
- 1 tablespoon vanilla

DIRECTIONS

1. Blend milk and eggs
2. In a pot sauté cauliflower for 2-3 minutes
3. Add the milk mixture and bring to simmer
4. Add vanilla, cinnamon, raisins
5. When ready remove and serve

Serves: **4**
Prep Time: **10**   Minutes
Cook Time: **20**   Minutes
Total Time: **30**   Minutes

INGREDIENTS

- ½ cup diced onion
- 2 cups rutabaga
- ½ tsp salt
- pepper

DIRECTIONS

1. In a frying pan add butter and sauté onion for 1-2 minutes
2. Add rutabaga, pepper, salt and continue cooking for another 8-9 minutes
3. Cook for another 4-5 minutes and remove rutabaga hash brown onto a plate and serve

Serves: *4*

Prep Time: *10*   Minutes

Cook Time: *30*   Minutes

Total Time: *40*   Minutes

INGREDIENTS

- 5 eggs
- 2 tablespoons butter
- 3 oz. wild salmon
- 3 scallions
- 2 tablespoons parsley
- 1 tablespoon dill
- salt

DIRECTIONS

1. Slice the scallions
2. Beat the eggs together
3. In a skillet heat butter and add the eggs
4. Add the remaining ingredients and mix well
5. Remove and serve

Serves: *3*
Prep Time: *5*   Minutes

Cook Time: *5*   Minutes

Total Time: *10*   Minutes

INGREDIENTS

- 2 eggs
- ½ cup pumpkin puree GAPS
- ¼ tsp cinnamon
- 1 tablespoon coconut oil
- honey

DIRECTIONS

1. Warm a cast iron over medium heat
2. Mix cinnamon, eggs, and pumpkin puree
3. Add coconut oil to the pan to the pan and pour pumpkin batter
4. Cook until golden brown
5. Remove and serve

Serves: **6**

Prep Time: **10** Minutes

Cook Time: **20** Minutes

Total Time: **30** Minutes

INGREDIENTS

- 3 eggs
- ½ cup coconut milk
- ½ tsp salt
- 1 tablespoon coconut flour

DIRECTIONS

1. Preheat your oven to 400 F
2. In a bowl mix all the ingredients
3. Fill muffin liners about 2/3 with batter
4. Bake for 15-20 minutes
5. Remove and serve

Serves: **2**
Prep Time: **10**   Minutes

Cook Time: **20**   Minutes

Total Time: **30**   Minutes

INGREDIENTS

- 4 cups squash
- ¼ cup butter
- 4 apples
- ¼ cup honey
- 1 tsp ginger
- 1 tablespoon almond flour

DIRECTIONS

1. Sauté the squash over medium heat
2. Add apples and sauté for another 1-2 minutes
3. Add in ginger, coconut flour, honey, and stir over medium heat for 4-5 minutes
4. Remove and serve

Serves: **2**

Prep Time: **10**   Minutes

Cook Time: **20**   Minutes

Total Time: **30**   Minutes

INGREDIENTS

- 2 tablespoons almond flour
- 2 tsp grassed gelatin(GAPS legal)
- ½ cup mashed butternut squash
- 2 tablespoons butter
- 2 eggs
- ½ tsp salt

DIRECTIONS

1. Preheat oven to 375 and line a baking sheet with parchment paper
2. Stir together the almond flour, gelatin, squash and butter
3. Stir in coconut flour, eggs, salt, and mix well
4. Spoon into rounds on the baking sheet and bake for 12-15 minutes or until ready

Serves: *2*
Prep Time: *5*   Minutes

Cook Time: *10*   Minutes

Total Time: *15*   Minutes

INGREDIENTS

- 2 egg whites
- ½ tsp almond flour
- additional seasonings

DIRECTIONS

1. Blend all ingredients until smooth
2. In a skillet pour the mixture and cook for 2-3 minutes
3. Remove and let wrap chill
4. Add seasoning and different ingredients to the wrap and serve (asparagus, chicken, fried potatoes)

Serves: **2**

Prep Time: **5**   Minutes

Cook Time: **5**   Minutes

Total Time: **10** Minutes

INGREDIENTS

- 1 lb. white bait
- 2 eggs
- 1 clove garlic
- herb

DIRECTIONS

1. In a bowl mix all ingredients
2. Pour mixture in a skillet and fry until golden on each side
3. Remove and serve

Serves: *4*
Prep Time: *10* Minutes

Cook Time: *30* Minutes

Total Time: *40* Minutes

INGREDIENTS

- 1 cup
- butter
- ½ cup honey
- 4 eggs
- 2 cups almond flour
- 1 tablespoon baking soda
- ¼ tablespoon salt
- 2 tablespoons cardamom
- ¼ cup berries
- ½ cup cherries
- ¼ cup raisins

DIRECTIONS

1. In a bowl mix honey, butter, eggs, and butter
2. Add baking soda cardamom, almond flour and fruits

3. Cook at 275 F for 40-45 minutes, remove and serve

LUNCH

CHERRY ORANGE SALAD

Serves: **2**

Prep Time: **5**   Minutes

Cook Time: **5**   Minutes

Total Time: **10** Minutes

INGREDIENTS

- 3 cups greens
- 3 oranges
- 1 cup cherries
- 2 tablespoons olive oil
- 2 tablespoons balsamic vinegar(SCD safe vinegar)

DIRECTIONS

1. Place greens, cherries, and orange in a bowl
2. Drizzle olive oil and vinegar and mix well
3. Serve when ready

Serves: *2*
Prep Time: *5*   Minutes

Cook Time: *5*   Minutes

Total Time: *10* Minutes

INGREDIENTS

- 1 roasted chicken
- ½ cup olive oil mayo
- ½ cup cilantro
- 1 head of butter lettuce
- 1 onion
- 1 lemon
- salt

DIRECTIONS

1. Shred the chicken and place it in a bowl
2. Add mayo, onion, cilantro, onion, salt, and pepper and mix well
3. Serve when ready

Serves: **2**

Prep Time: **5** Minutes

Cook Time: **5** Minutes

Total Time: **10** Minutes

INGREDIENTS

- 2 carrots
- 1 cup peas
- 1 cup cabbage
- ¼ cucumber
- 1 cup mango
- 1 tablespoons hazelnuts
- ½ cup chicken breast meat
- ½ cup salad dressing
- 1 tablespoon cilantro

DIRECTIONS

1. In a bowl place all salad ingredients
2. Drizzle salad dressing over salad and mix well
3. Serve when ready

CUCUMBER SALAD

Serves: **2**

Prep Time: **5**   Minutes

Cook Time: **5**   Minutes

Total Time: **10** Minutes

INGREDIENTS

- 1 cucumber
- 1 tsp salt
- 3 green onions
- 2 tablespoons cilantro
- ½ cup lemon juice
- ½ cup olive oil
- 1 tsp lemon zest
- ¼ tsp pepper

DIRECTIONS

1. Slice cucumber
2. Slice green onions, add chop cilantro and lemon zest
3. Mix onions, lemon juice, lemon zest, olive oil, cilantro, cracked pepper
4. Pour dressing over the salad and serve

Serves: *2*

Prep Time: *5*   Minutes

Cook Time: *5*   Minutes

Total Time: *10*   Minutes

INGREDIENTS

- 3 cups lettuce mixed varieties
- 1 cup cooked chicken
- 2 boiled eggs
- ½ cup sunflower seeds
- ½ cup salad dressing

DIRECTIONS

1. In a bowl pour all salad ingredients
2. Drizzle salad dressing over and mix well
3. Serve when ready

Serves: *2*
Prep Time: *5*   Minutes

Cook Time: *5*   Minutes

Total Time: *10*   Minutes

INGREDIENTS

- 10 oz. tuna fish
- ¼ cup mayo
- 1 rib celery
- 1 carrot
- 1 shallot
- 1 tablespoon dill
- 1 tablespoon lemon juice
-

DIRECTIONS

1. **In a bowl mix all ingredients**
2. **Serve with salad dressing**

Serves: **2**

Prep Time: **5** Minutes

Cook Time: **5** Minutes

Total Time: **10** Minutes

INGREDIENTS

- 1 cup arugula
- 2 Campari cocktails
- ¼ avocado pitted
- 2 sliced mozzarella cheese
- basil leaves
- 1 tablespoon olive oil
- 1 tsp balsamic vinegar(SCD Safe vinegar)
- salt

DIRECTIONS

1. In a bowl mix avocado, mozzarella, tomato
2. Top with basil leaves
3. Whisk olive oil with balsamic vinegar, honey, and sugar
4. Toss to coat and serve

Serves: **2**
Prep Time: **5**   Minutes

Cook Time: **5**   Minutes

Total Time: **10**   Minutes

INGREDIENTS

- 3 chicken breasts
- 1 onion
- 1 yellow bell pepper
- 2 heads romaine hearts
- 1 avocado
- 1/3 cup cherry tomatoes

MARINADE

- ¼ cup cilantro
- 1 lime
- 1 tsp salt
- 1 clove garlic
- 1 tsp cumin
- 1 tsp chili powder
- ½ cup olive oil

DIRECTIONS

1. In a blender place all ingredients and blend until smooth
2. Pour marinade over and refrigerate

TOMATO AVOCADO SALAD

Serves: *2*
Prep Time: *5*   Minutes

Cook Time: *5*   Minutes

Total Time: *10*   Minutes

INGREDIENTS

- 1 lb. tomatoes
- 1 cucumber
- ¼ onion sliced
- 1 avocados
- 1 tablespoon olive oil
- 1 tablespoon lemon juice
- ½ cup cilantro
- 1 tsp salt
- ¼ tsp black pepper

DIRECTIONS

1. Place all ingredients in a bowl
2. Drizzle olive oil, lemon juice
3. Toss to combine and serve

Serves: *4*
Prep Time: *5*   Minutes

Cook Time: *5*   Minutes

Total Time: *10*   Minutes

INGREDIENTS

- ½ cup onion
- ½ cup lime juice
- 3 cups watermelon
- ½ cup cheddar cheese
- ¼ tsp pepper
- ½ cup cilantro

DIRECTIONS

1. Soak the onion in the lime juice
2. Combine all ingredients into a bowl
3. Serve when ready

Serves: **12**

Prep Time: **10** Minutes

Cook Time: **90** Minutes

Total Time: **100** Minutes

INGREDIENTS

- 1 chicken
- coconut oil
- 1 onion
- 3 cups rhubarb
- 3 cloves garlic
- 1-inch ginger
- 1 tablespoon coriander
- 10 vegetables

DIRECTIONS

1. In a pot add giblets, chicken, and cover with water
2. Bring to boil and cook for 60 minutes, heat a cast iron pan over medium heat
3. Add coconut oil, onion, rhubarb and sauté for 10-12 minutes

4. Add ginger, spices, garlic, stir in and sauté for 2-3 minutes

5. Remove chicken from pot and place on a plate

6. Add rhubarb mixture and vegetables into the soup and simmer for 25-30 minutes

7. Add chicken back, stir to combine and serve

Serves: *8*

Prep Time: *10*   Minutes

Cook Time: *180*   Minutes

Total Time: *190*   Minutes

INGREDIENTS

- 1 package grass fed
- 1 package marrow bones
- 1 cup water
- 10 cup chopped vegetables

DIRECTIONS

1. Place soup and marrow bones into a pot and cover with water
2. Bring to boil and let it simmer for 2-3 hours
3. Add vegetables to the broth and bring to simmer for 25-30 minutes
4. Add marrow fat and place meat in the blender and blend until smooth
5. Remove meat from the blender and add to the cooked vegetables

Serves: **6**
Prep Time: **20**   Minutes

Cook Time: **35**   Minutes

Total Time: **55**   Minutes

INGREDIENTS

- 3 tablespoons sesame oil
- 3-inch ginger
- 15 garlic cloves
- 1 tsp black pepper
- 1 pinch ground cloves
- 2 tablespoons coconut aminos
- 1 tablespoon fish sauce
- 1 tablespoon honey
- 1 cup basil leaves

DIRECTIONS

1. In a skillet add sesame oil over medium heat
2. Add garlic, pepper, ginger, cloves and sauté for 2-3 minutes
3. Add chicken and cook for 5-10 minutes

4. Add honey, fish sauce, coconut aminos and bring to boil

5. Simmer for 12-15 minutes, remove from heat, add basil leaves and serve

ITALIAN VEGETABLE SOUP

Serves: **4**

Prep Time: **10** Minutes

Cook Time: **30** Minutes

Total Time: **40** Minutes

INGREDIENTS

- 2 tablespoons butter
- ¼ onion
- 2 carrots
- 2 stalks celery
- 4 cup chicken broth
- 10 oz. frozen cauliflower
- 1 cup green beans
- 28 oz. can tomatoes

- 2 tsp basil leaves
- 2 tsp oregano
- 2 tsp garlic powder
- 1 tsp salt
- ¼ black pepper

DIRECTIONS

1. **Melt the butter into a pot**
2. **Saute carrots, celery, onions for 4-5 minutes**
3. **Reduce heat and add the rest of ingredients and simmer for 15-20 minutes**
4. **Remove from heat, add cheese and serve**

CARROT SOUP

Serves: *8*
Prep Time: *10*   Minutes

Cook Time: *30*   Minutes

Total Time: *40*   Minutes

INGREDIENTS

- 16-18 carrots
- 6 cups
- 2 onions
- 2-inch ginger root
- 2-inch turmeric root
- 2 tablespoons coconut oil
- 2 tablespoons apple cider vinegar(SCD Safe vinegar)
- ¼ tsp salt
- ¼ tsp black pepper

DIRECTIONS

1. In a pot heat chicken broth over medium heat
2. Peel carrots, chop carrots, onion, turmeric, ginger root and add them to the broth
3. Add salt and simmer for 18-20 minutes
4. Blend everything until smooth and serve

Serves: *6*
Prep Time: *10*   Minutes

Cook Time: *20*   Minutes

Total Time: *30*   Minutes

INGREDIENTS

- 1 tablespoon butter
- 1 onion
- 1 garlic clove
- 1 cup celery root
- 2 cups homemade broth
- 1 tsp dried dill
- 6 oz. sausage

DIRECTIONS

1. In a saucepan melt butter, add garlic onion and sauté for 4-5 minutes
2. Add broth, celery root and bring to boil
3. Reduce heat and simmer for 15-20 minutes
4. Blend everything until smooth and transfer back to the pot

5. Add dill, sausage and cook on low heat until ready
6. Remove and serve

CHICKEN POT SOUP

Serves: *4*
Prep Time: *10*   Minutes

Cook Time: *30*   Minutes

Total Time: *40*   Minutes

INGREDIENTS

- ¼ tablespoons butter
- 1 onion
- ¼ celery root
- 4 cups chicken broth
- ½ cup coconut milk
- 2 carrots
- 2 tsp salt
- ½ tsp black pepper
- 1 lb. cooked chicken
- 1/3 cup peas

- 1 tsp fresh thyme
- ¼ tsp rosemary

DIRECTIONS

1. In a saucepan heat butter over medium heat and add onions
2. Add celery root and broth, bring to boil for 8-10 minutes
3. Remove celery root and blend it with coconut milk
4. Add it back to the saucepan with carrots, pepper, herbs and simmer for 12-15 minutes
5. Stir in chicken, peas and serve when ready

BASIL SOUP

Serves:	*4*	
Prep Time:	*10*	Minutes
Cook Time:	*30*	Minutes
Total Time:	*40*	Minutes

INGREDIENTS

51

- 2 tablespoons butter
- ¼ onion
- 1 carrot
- 1 lb. tomatoes
- 2 cup homemade chicken
- 2 tablespoons dried basil
- ¼ tsp salt
- ¼ tsp pepper

DIRECTIONS

1. In a saucepan melt butter, add carrot, onion and sauté for 4-5 minutes
2. Add beef broth, tomatoes, salt, basil and simmer for 15-20 minutes
3. Cool and blend mixture until smooth
4. Pour into bowls and serve

TURKEY SOUP

Serves: *4*
Prep Time: *10* Minutes

Cook Time: *35* Minutes

Total Time: *45* Minutes

INGREDIENTS

- 2-quarts turkey stock
- 2 beets
- 1 onion
- 3 carrots
- 2 cups peas
- 2 cups green beans
- ¼ head cabbage
- 8 Swiss chard leaves
- 2 cups cooked turkey meat

DIRECTIONS

1. In a pot add turkey stock, beets, greens, onions and cook over medium heat
2. Add carrots, peas, green beans, cabbage, Swiss chars leaves and bring to boil

3. Simmer for about 30 minutes, add turkey meat and simmer for another 5-10 minutes

4. Remove from heat and serve

CAULIFLOWER SOUP

Serves: *4*
Prep Time: *10*   Minutes

Cook Time: *30*   Minutes

Total Time: *40*   Minutes

INGREDIENTS

- ½ onion
- 2 tablespoons coconut
- 1-quart chicken stock
- 1-quart water
- 1 head cauliflower
- 5 sausages
- 2 cups coconut milk
- 2 tablespoons minced garlic
- 1 tablespoon oregano

- ¼ tablespoon sage
- ½ tablespoon paprika
- salt

DIRECTIONS

1. In a pot add onion, oil and sauté over medium heat for 8-10 minutes
2. Add cauliflower to the pot, cover with stock and water and bring to boil
3. Cook until cauliflower is tender and add sausage and remaining ingredients
4. When ready remove from heat and serve

ZUCCHINI CHIPS

Serves: *4*

Prep Time: *5*   Minutes

Cook Time: *10*   Hours

Total Time: *10*   Hours *5* Minutes

INGREDIENTS

- 1 lb. zucchini
- 1 tablespoon oil
- 1 tsp salt

DIRECTIONS

1. Slice zucchini into thin slices
2. Toss in salt and oil
3. Arrange in a single on a dehydrator tray
4. Dehydrate at 125 F for 10-12 hours
5. When ready remove and serve

Serves: *4*

Prep Time: *10*   Minutes

Cook Time: *7*   Hours

Total Time: *7*   Hours and 10 Minutes

INGREDIENTS

- 1 tablespoon butter
- 2 lbs. beef roast
- 1 onion
- 6 cloves garlic
- 3 slices bacon
- ¼ cup red wine
- ½ tsp rosemary
- ¼ tsp dried thyme
- pinch of salt

DIRECTIONS

1. In a skillet heat butter, add beef roast and brown on all sides, remove and place to a crock pot
2. Sauté onions, bacon, garlic and move to crock pot
3. Add onion, seasoning and cook on low for 6-7 hours

Serves: **2**

Prep Time: **10**   Minutes

Cook Time: **50**   Minutes

Total Time: **60**   Minutes

INGREDIENTS

- 1 squash
- 1 onion
- 2 cup leftover turkey
- 2 apples
- 1 cup cranberries
- 1 tsp cinnamon
- 1 tsp salt
- ¼ tsp nutmeg
- ¼ cup butter

DIRECTIONS

1. Preheat oven to 325 F
2. Cut squash in half and slice into half rings and place in a bowl
3. Toss with spices, cranberries, apples

4. Pour into baking dish and bake for 40-50 minutes or until tender

5. Remove and serve

PARMESAN DRUMSTICKS

Serves: *3*
Prep Time: *10* Minutes

Cook Time: *40* Minutes

Total Time: *50* Minutes

INGREDIENTS

- 2 eggs
- 2 cups parmesan cheese
- 1 tsp salt
- 1 tsp black pepper
- 12 chicken drumsticks
- coconut oil

DIRECTIONS

1. Preheat oven to 375 F
2. In a bowl crack eggs, beat them and set aside
3. In another bowl mix cheese, pepper, salt and set aside
4. Dip the drumsticks into the eggs mixture and coat evenly
5. Roll into cheese mixture and place in the baking pan
6. Bake for 40-50 minutes, remove and serve

SWEDISH MEATBALLS

Serves: **6**

Prep Time: **10** Minutes

Cook Time: **20** Minutes

Total Time: **30** Minutes

INGREDIENTS

- 1 cup sunflower oil
- ¼ cup coconut milk
- 1 tsp onion powder
- 1 tsp
- salt
- 4 lbs. ground beef
-
- 2 eggs
- 1 tsp black pepper
- ¼ tsp allspice
- ¼ tsp nutmeg

SAUCE

- ½ cup butter
- ¼ cup parmesan cheese
- 5 cups beef broth

- ¼ cup coconut milk
- salt

DIRECTIONS

1. Preheat oven to 375 F
2. In a bowl mix all meatballs ingredients using a stand mixer
3. Form little balls and bake for 20-25 minutes or until done
4. In a skillet sauce parmesan cheese, whisk in beef broth, salt, and coconut milk, cook until thickened
5. Serve on top of meatballs

ZUCCHINI LASAGNA

Serves: **6**

Prep Time: **10** Minutes

Cook Time: **20** Minutes

Total Time: **30** Minutes

INGREDIENTS

- 1 onion
- 3 cloves garlic
- 2 tablespoon butter
- 1 lb. ground beef
- 1 lb. Italian sausage
- 1 tablespoon oregano
- ¼ cup basil
- ¼ tsp cayenne pepper
- salt
- 14 oz. can diced tomatoes
- 6 oz. can tomato paste
- 4 zucchinis
- 3 cup cheddar cheese

DIRECTIONS

1. Preheat oven to 325 F
2. Slice the zucchinis into long strips
3. In a pot sauté the onions and garlic
4. Add Italian sausage, beef, basil, cayenne, pepper, oregano and cook for 5-6 minutes
5. Add tomato paste and tomatoes and cook for another 4-5 minutes
6. Bake for 40-45 minutes, remove and serve

Serves: **4**

Prep Time: **10** Minutes

Cook Time: **30** Minutes

Total Time: **40** Minutes

INGREDIENTS

- 2 acorn squash
- ¼ cup butter
- ½ cup shallots
- 2 apples
- ¼ tsp salt
- ½ tsp black pepper
- ¼ tsp cinnamon
- ½ tsp nutmeg

DIRECTIONS

1. Preheat oven to 325 F
2. Bake squash for 20-25 minutes
3. Sauté the shallots until tender, add salt, pepper, apples, nutmeg, and cinnamon

4. Fill each squash with apple mixture, bake for 25-30 minutes
5. Remove and serve

Serves: *2*

Prep Time: *10*   Minutes

Cook Time: *20*   Minutes

Total Time: *30*   Minutes

INGREDIENTS

- 2 lbs. ground chicken
- 2 onions
- 3 garlic cloves
- 1 yellow squash
- 1 bell pepper
- 1 bunch basil
- salt
- 1 cup Italian dressing
- 1 head romaine lettuce

DIRECTIONS

1. Cook ground chicken until tender with garlic, pepper, basil, onions, and squash
2. Serve the squash with lettuce leaves and Italian dressing

Serves: *2*
Prep Time: *10*   Minutes

Cook Time: *20*   Minutes

Total Time: *30*   Minutes

INGREDIENTS

- 2 tablespoons sesame oil
- 2-inch piece ginger
- 16-18 garlic cloves
- 1 tsp black pepper
- 1 pinch cloves
- 1,5 lbs. chicken drumsticks
- 2 tablespoons coconut aminos
- 1 tablespoon fish sauce
- 1 tablespoon honey
- 1 cup basil leaves

DIRECTIONS

1. **In a skillet add sesame oil, pepper, cloves, garlic, ginger and sauté for 3-4 minutes**

2. Add chicken and cook for 6-7 minutes, add honey coconut aminos, fish sauce and bring to boil
3. Lower the heat and simmer for 14-16 minutes
4. Add basil, stir to combine and serve when ready

SPAGHETTI WITH MEATBALLS

Serves: **12**
Prep Time: **10** Minutes

Cook Time: **20** Minutes

Total Time: **30** Minutes

INGREDIENTS

- 3 zucchini
- 2 cups sauce
- 1 b. ground beef
- 1 onion
- 2 cloves garlic
- 1 tablespoon herbs
- 1 tablespoon butter

DIRECTIONS

1. Cook spaghetti squash and set aside

2. In a bowl mix garlic, seasoning, onion, ground beef, and divide into 12-14 meatballs

3. Add the meatballs into a pot and cook until they are browned

4. Add sauce, seasoning and simmer for 10-12 minutes

5. Add vegetable noodles cook until done and remove from heat

6. Add salt and serve

Serves: **6**

Prep Time: **10**   Minutes

Cook Time: **50**   Minutes

Total Time: **60**   Minutes

INGREDIENTS

- 2 lbs. chicken pieces drumsticks
- ½ cup parmesan cheese
- 2 tablespoons almond flour
- 1 tsp garlic powder
- 1 tsp dried basil 1 tsp salt
- black pepper
- 2 heads broccoli

DIRECTIONS

1. Preheat oven to 350 F
2. Lay chicken in a pan and sprinkle with garlic powder, parmesan basil, pepper and salt
3. Add 2 tablespoons butter and bake for 40-45 minutes
4. Remove from oven and transfer to a plate
5. Serve with baked broccoli

Serves: **2**

Prep Time: **5**   Minutes

Cook Time: **5**   Minutes

Total Time: **10**   Minutes

INGREDIENTS

- 1 cup c
- oconut milk
- ½ cup gelatin (SCD Safe)
- 6 oz. cheddar cheese
- ¼ tsp salt

DIRECTIONS

1. In a saucepan heat milk and stir occasionally
2. Chop cheese into small chunks and place cheese in a blender
3. Add the milk and blend for 20-30 seconds
4. Pour into saucepan and lower heat
5. When ready remove and serve

Serves: *4*

Prep Time: *10*   Minutes

Cook Time: *30*   Minutes

Total Time: *40*   Minutes

INGREDIENTS

- 3 mushrooms
- 3 oz. tomato paste
- 2 tablespoons avocado oil
- ¼ salt
- ¼ tsp dried basil
- 1 clove garlic

DIRECTIONS

1. Preheat oven to 375 F
2. In a skillet add chopped mushrooms, garlic, basil and sauté for 2-3 minutes, transfer to a bowl
3. Add tomato paste and stir well
4. Fill each cavity of mushrooms with tomato paste and place into baking pan
5. Top with meat, cheese, olives and bake for 20-25 minutes

Serves: *4*
Prep Time: *10*   Minutes

Cook Time: *70*   Minutes

Total Time: *80*   Minutes

INGREDIENTS

- 2 lbs. zucchini
- 3 cups bone broth
- 1 cup chorizo
- 2 bell peppers
- 5 tablespoons butter

DIRECTIONS

1. Cut zucchini into ½ inch slices and place in a saucepan
2. Add bone broth and simmer for 25-30 minutes
3. Add peppers, chorizo and simmer for another 20 minutes
4. Stir in stew, butter and cook for another 10-12 minutes
5. Remove from heat and serve when ready

TARRAGON ZUCCHINI

Serves: **4**

Prep Time: **5** Minutes

Cook Time: **15** Minutes

Total Time: **20** Minutes

INGREDIENTS

- ¼ tablespoon butter
- 1 zucchini
- 1 tablespoon tarragon leaves
- ½ cup heavy cream

DIRECTIONS

1. In a pan melt butter over medium heat
2. Sauté the zucchini for 6-7 minutes, add tarragon and cook until tender
3. Remove and serve

Serves: *4*

Prep Time: *10*   Minutes

Cook Time: *30*   Minutes

Total Time: *40*   Minutes

INGREDIENTS

- 1 onion
- 1 carrot
- 2 tablespoons lard
- 1 cup lentils
- 13 oz. organic almond milk
- 1 tsp cinnamon
- 1 tsp cumin
- 1 tsp turmeric
- 1tsp thyme
- 6 roasted garlic cloves
- 1 pinch red pepper flakes
- 1 cup kale

DIRECTIONS

1. In a pot melt butter over medium heat, add onion and carrots
2. Add garlic, lentils, veggies, and stir
3. Add almond milk, spices, stock and simmer for 25-30 minutes
4. Add kale and simmer for a couple of more minutes before removing from heat

WHITE BEAN CHILI

Serves: *4*

Prep Time: *10*   Minutes

Cook Time: *30*   Minutes

Total Time: *40*   Minutes

INGREDIENTS

- 2 lb. ground beef
-
- 1 onion
- 1 tsp garlic powder

- 2-quarts chicken broth
- 1 cup almond milk
-
- 1 tsp salt
- ¼ tsp black pepper
- 1 tablespoon cumin powder
- 1 tsp paprika

DIRECTIONS

1. Brown the meat with diced onion
2. Add the rest of ingredients and simmer for 25-30 minutes
3. When ready, remove from heat and serve

Serves: *2*

Prep Time: *10*   Minutes

Cook Time: *15*   Minutes

Total Time: *25*   Minutes

INGREDIENTS

- 1 head cauliflower
- 1-quart homemade stock
- 1 tsp sat
- ½ cup butter

DIRECTIONS

1. Boil cauliflower in stock until tender
2. In a blender add salt, butter and blend until smooth
3. When ready remove and serve

Serves: *4*
Prep Time: *10*   Minutes

Cook Time: *4*   Hours

Total Time: *4*   Hours and 10 Minutes

INGREDIENTS

- 1 pasture-raised duck
- ½ cup butter
- 1 pinch salt
- 1 onion
- 1 cup white wine

DIRECTIONS

1. Rinse the duck and pat it dry
2. Spread butter over the duck breast
3. Stuff the duck's cavity with onion and pour wine into the roasting pan and place the duck in the pan
4. Bake for 4 hours at 350 F or until tender
5. Remove and serve with cherry sauce

Serves: **8**

Prep Time: **10** Minutes

Cook Time: **50** Minutes

Total Time: **60** Minutes

INGREDIENTS
- 5 slices bacon
- 1 onion
- ¼ tsp salt
- ¼ tsp black pepper
- 1 bunch broccoli
- 1 cup cheddar cheese

DIRECTIONS

1. Preheat oven to 375
2. In a skillet add bacon and cook until crispy
3. Add onion and cook until golden brown
4. In a bowl beat eggs, salt, pepper and add broccoli on top and bake for 20 minutes
5. Remove, slice into wedges and serve

GUMMY BEARS

Serves: **4**

Prep Time: **10**   Minutes

Cook Time: **30**   Minutes

Total Time: **40**   Minutes

INGREDIENTS

- ½ cup hot water
- 2 tablespoon gelatin
- 1 tablespoon cocoa powder
- 1 tablespoon honey
- 1 pinch salt

DIRECTIONS

1. In a skillet heat water and add gelatin
2. Add honey, cocoa powder, salt and whisk until completely mixed
3. Pour mixture into a silicone mold, place in the freezer for 15-20 minutes
4. Remove and serve

Serves: **12**

Prep Time: **10** Minutes

Cook Time: **15** Minutes

Total Time: **25** Minutes

INGREDIENTS

- ½ coconut oil
- ½ cup honey
- ¼ tsp salt
- ¼ tablespoon baking soda
- 2 tablespoons vanilla extract
- 1 cup almond flour
- 1 egg

DIRECTIONS

1. Preheat oven to 300 F
2. In a bowl mix all ingredients using a hand mixer
3. Scoop balls of dough and bake for 10-15 minutes
4. Remove, allow to cool and serve

Serves: **4**

Prep Time: **10**   Minutes

Cook Time: **30**   Minutes

Total Time: **40**   Minutes

INGREDIENTS

- 2 tablespoons powdered gelatin
- ¼ cup water
- 4 egg yolks
- 5 tablespoons honey
- 1 tablespoon vanilla extract
- 5 chocolate almond flour

DIRECTIONS

1. In hot water add powdered gelatin and mix well
2. In a pan add egg yolk, honey and whisk well
3. Whisk for 6-7 minutes, remove from heat and allow to cool
4. Refrigerate for 5-6 hours, when chilled, add to your ice cream maker
5. Remove form small cookies and serve

Serves: *6*
Prep Time: *10*   Minutes

Cook Time: *10*   Minutes

Total Time: *20*   Minutes

INGREDIENTS

- 5 eggs
- 1 banana
- 1 tablespoon vanilla
- ¼ cup almond flour
- ¼ tsp cinnamon
- ½ tsp cloves
- ¼ tsp baking soda

DIRECTIONS

1. In a blender add vanilla, eggs, bananas, baking soda, spices, almond flour, and blend until smooth
2. Spoon ¼ cup into the middle of your griddle
3. Bake for 1-2 minutes per side
4. Remove and serve with topping

Serves: **3**

Prep Time: **10** Minutes

Cook Time: **30** Minutes

Total Time: **40** Minutes

INGREDIENTS

- ½ cup coconut cream
- ½ cup coconut oil
- 1 tablespoon vanilla
- 2 tablespoons honey
- ¼ cup pecans
- 2 tablespoons butter
- ¼ cup shredded coconut

DIRECTIONS

1. Butter a container and place a parchment paper
2. Stir in coconut cream concentrate
3. Mix all ingredients together, and spread the fudge into the container
4. Freeze for 20-30 minutes
5. Remove and serve

Serves: **4**

Prep Time: **10** Minutes

Cook Time: **30** Minutes

Total Time: **40** Minutes

INGREDIENTS

- 3 cups almond flour
- ¼ cup honey
- 1 egg
- 1 tablespoon vanilla
- ¼ tsp salt
- ¾ cup butter
- 1 cup peanut butter
- ½ cup honey

DIRECTIONS

1. In a bowl mix all dry ingredients
2. In another bowl mix all wet ingredients and pour over dry ingredients and mix well
3. Spoon into small cookies and bake at 325 F for 10-15 minutes

Serves: **6**

Prep Time: **10** Minutes

Cook Time: **20** Minutes

Total Time: **30** Minutes

INGREDIENTS

- 5 tablespoons coconut flour
- ¼ tsp salt
- ¼ tsp baking soda
- 4 eggs
- ¼ cup butter
- ½ cup honey
- 1 tsp vanilla

DIRECTIONS

1. Place all ingredients in a bowl and blend using a hand mixer
2. Pour butter into a cupcake tin and dust with coconut flour
3. Bake at 300 F for 20-25 minutes, remove and serve

Serves: *4*
Prep Time: *10*   Minutes

Cook Time: *30*   Minutes

Total Time: *40*   Minutes

INGREDIENTS

- 1 cup coconut cream
- 1 tablespoon honey
- 1 tablespoon butter

DIRECTIONS

1. In a bowl mix honey and butter
2. Remove the coconut cream from the can and place in a bowl
3. Whip with a mixer, chill and serve

Serves: **6**

Prep Time: **10** Minutes

Cook Time: **20** Minutes

Total Time: **30** Minutes

INGREDIENTS

- 1 cup raw cashews
- ¼ cup almonds

1/2 cup almond flour
- ½ cup coconut oil
- 2 tablespoons honey
- 1 cup shredded coconut
- 1 tsp vanilla
- 1 pinch salt

DIRECTIONS

1. Soak cashews for a couple of hours
2. Preheat oven to 325 F
3. In a bowl mix, almond flour with baking soda and mix will wet ingredients
4. Pour batter into a pan and bake for 20 minutes

Serves: *1*

Prep Time: 5   Minutes

Cook Time: 5   Minutes

Total Time: *10*   Minutes

INGREDIENTS

- 1 cup coconut milk
- 1 handful spinach leaves
- 1 avocado
- 1 tablespoon vanilla extract
- 1 cup ice cubes
- 2
- spearmint leaves

DIRECTIONS

1. In a blender place all ingredients and blend until smooth
2. Pour smoothie in a glass and serve

Serves: *1*

Prep Time: *5*   Minutes

Cook Time: *5*   Minutes

Total Time: *10*   Minutes

INGREDIENTS

- 1 banana
- ½ cup coconut milk
- 1 tsp vanilla
- ½ tsp cinnamon powder
- 1 tablespoon peanut butter
- 2 crushed ice cubes
- 1 egg yolk

DIRECTIONS

1. In a blender place all ingredients and blend until smooth
2. Pour smoothie in a glass and serve

Serves: **1**

Prep Time: **5** Minutes

Cook Time: **5** Minutes

Total Time: **10** Minutes

INGREDIENTS

- 2 cups cooked carrots
- 1 cup raw milk
- ¼ cup heavy grass-fed cream
- 2 scoops collagen peptides
- 1-inch turmeric
- 1-inch ginger
- ½ tsp cinnamon

DIRECTIONS

1. In a blender place all ingredients and blend until smooth
2. Pour smoothie in a glass and serve

Serves: *1*

Prep Time: *5* Minutes

Cook Time: *5* Minutes

Total Time: *10* Minutes

INGREDIENTS

- 1 cup juice
- 1 raw egg
- 1 tablespoons butter

DIRECTIONS

1. In a blender place all ingredients and blend until smooth
2. Pour smoothie in a glass and serve

Serves: *1*

Prep Time: *5*   Minutes

Cook Time: *5*   Minutes

Total Time: *10*   Minutes

INGREDIENTS

- 1 avocado
- 1 banana
- ½ cup coconut oil
- ¼ cup peanut butter
- 1 scoop protein powder
- ½ cup homemade SCD yogurt
- ¼ cup kefir

DIRECTIONS

1. In a blender place all ingredients and blend until smooth
2. Pour smoothie in a glass and serve

Serves: **1**

Prep Time: **5** Minutes

Cook Time: **5** Minutes

Total Time: **10** Minutes

INGREDIENTS

- 2 bananas
- 1 tablespoon coconut flakes
- 1 cup milk
-
- 1 tablespoon peanut butter

DIRECTIONS

1. In a blender place all ingredients and blend until smooth
2. Pour smoothie in a glass and serve

Serves: *1*

Prep Time: *5*   Minutes

Cook Time: *5*   Minutes

Total Time: *10*   Minutes

INGREDIENTS

- 1 cup almond milk
- 1 banana
- 1 tsp pure vanilla extract
- 8 ice cubes

DIRECTIONS

1. In a blender place all ingredients and blend until smooth
2. Pour smoothie in a glass and serve

Serves: *1*

Prep Time: *5*   Minutes

Cook Time: *5*   Minutes

Total Time: *10* Minutes

INGREDIENTS

- 12 chai tea ice cubes
- 2 cups milk
- 1/2 cup
- coconut flakes
- whipped cream

DIRECTIONS

1. In a blender place all ingredients and blend until smooth
2. Pour smoothie in a glass and serve

Serves: *1*
Prep Time: *5*   Minutes

Cook Time: *5*   Minutes

Total Time: *10*   Minutes

INGREDIENTS

- 10 pitted dates
- ½ cup almonds
- 1/2 c
- up coffee
- ¼ cup almond breeze
- 5 ice cubes

DIRECTIONS

1. In a blender place all ingredients and blend until smooth
2. Pour smoothie in a glass and serve

VEGAN SMOOTHIE

Serves: **1**

Prep Time: **5**   Minutes

Cook Time: **5**   Minutes

Total Time: **10**   Minutes

INGREDIENTS

- 2 bananas
- 5 ice cubes
- 1 tablespoon coconut oil
- 1 tablespoon diary free yogurt(SCD safe)
- 1 tablespoon chia seeds
- 1 tsp p
- rotein powder
-
- ½ cup coconut milk

DIRECTIONS

1. In a blender place all ingredients and blend until smooth
2. Pour smoothie in a glass and serve

Serves: *1*
Prep Time: *5*   Minutes
Cook Time: *5*   Minutes
Total Time: *10* Minutes

INGREDIENTS

- 10 oz. frozen raspberries
- ¼ cup vanilla kefir
- 1 tablespoon hemp
- 1 cup orange juice

DIRECTIONS

1. In a blender place all ingredients and blend until smooth
2. Pour smoothie in a glass and serve

THANK YOU FOR READING THIS BOOK!

Made in the USA
Middletown, DE
22 October 2023

41237212R00061